Outdoor Adventures and Energy Foods

Uniting Nature and Nutrition

Table of Contents

1. Introduction 1

2. Exploring the Great Outdoors: An Intriguing Prelude 2

   2.1. The Call of the Wild 2

   2.2. Facets of Outdoor Adventures 2

   2.3. The Essence of Adventure and the Role of Physical Fitness . . . 3

   2.4. Role of Mental Well-being 4

   2.5. Outdoor Adventures & Sustainable Tourism 4

3. The Importance of Nutrition in Outdoor Adventures 5

   3.1. Understanding the Connection 5

   3.2. The Role of Macronutrients 5

   3.3. Hydration is Key 6

   3.4. Meal Planning Strategies 6

   3.5. Wrapping it Up 7

4. Fueling the Adventure: A Look into Energy Foods 8

   4.1. The Energy Demand of Outdoor Activities 8

   4.2. Essential Nutrients for Outdoor Activities 8

   4.3. Favorite Energy Foods of Adventurers 9

   4.4. Energy Food Recipes for the Outdoors 10

      4.4.1. Energy Bars 10

      4.4.2. Peanut Butter Sandwich with a Twist 10

   4.5. H20: The Essential Element 10

   4.6. Beyond Nutrition 11

5. Matching the Terrain: Tailoring Nutrition to Adventure Types . . . 12

   5.1. Trekking in Mountains 12

   5.2. Canoeing and Kayaking 13

   5.3. Desert Exploration 13

   5.4. Rock Climbing 13

   5.5. Arctic Adventures 14

5.6. Jungle Safari 14

6. The Backpack Chef: Preparing Energy Foods in the Wild . . 16

6.1. Gathering Your Tools 16

6.2. Provisioning Creatively 17

6.3. Mastering the Art of Wild Cooking 17

6.4. Staying Hydrated 18

6.5. Cleanup and Waste Management 18

7. Eating on the Trail: Nutritious On-The-Go Meal Ideas 20

7.1. The Principles of Trail Nutrition 20

7.2. Healthful Meal Ideas for Hikers 21

7.3. Power Breakfasts 21

7.4. Mid-Trail Lunches 21

7.5. Sustaining Dinners 22

7.6. Energizing Snacks and Desserts 22

8. Foraging 101: Learning from Nature's Pantry 23

8.1. Digging into History 23

8.2. Essential Foraging skills 23

8.3. Safety & Preparation 24

8.4. Guided Foraging Adventure 24

8.5. Making Meals 24

8.6. The Bountiful Nutrition 25

8.7. Forage for a Cause 25

9. Food Safety: Keeping Your Outdoor Meals Fresh and Clean . . 26

9.1. Understanding Foodborne Illnesses 26

9.2. Kit Essentials: Storage and Cooking Devices 26

9.3. Safe Food Storage 27

9.4. Safe Water Storage 27

9.5. Meal Preparation in the Outdoors 28

9.6. Safe Trash Disposal 28

10. Case Studies: Thriving against Elements with the Right Fuel . . 29

10.1. First Case: Mike Leary, the Arctic Survivor 29

10.2. Second Case: Emma White, the Long-distance Swimmer . . . 30

10.3. Third Case: Max Li, the Desert Explorer 31

11. Embracing the Future: The Confluence of Adventure and Nutrition 33

11.1. The Enthralling Alliance 33

11.2. The Rise of Adventure Nutrition 34

11.3. The Science of Performance Foods 34

11.4. Fueling Up for Outdoor Challenges 35

11.5. Nourishing the Adventurer's Spirit 35

Chapter 1. Introduction

Take a dive into the invigorating world of outdoor adventures, where the verdant embrace of nature bids you welcome, with our special report: "Outdoor Adventures and Energy Foods: Uniting Nature and Nutrition". This report captures the delightful unity of challenging adventures under the open sky and the appetizing energy-packed foods that fuel them. Want to learn about the secrets of harnessing nature's bounty for nutritious on-the-go meals? Let's follow the trail. We promise to weave a tale of exploration across rugged terrains, canoeing on glistening lakes and trekking atop towering cliffs, all while maintaining a tandem with the nutritious fuel necessary for such exploits. This cheerful, buoyant journey will awaken the explorer within you, prompting you not only to discover more about the great outdoors, but to delve deeper into the wellspring of nutritional wisdom that sustains it. Come, it's time to chart an exciting path where nature's grandeur meets nutritional science!

Chapter 2. Exploring the Great Outdoors: An Intriguing Prelude

The journey starts here, with the dawn light just kissing the horizon, casting long shadows on the dew-kissed forest paths awaiting the eager tread of adventurers.

2.1. The Call of the Wild

The great outdoors has, since time immemorial, enticed mankind into its grand expanse, teasing the inherent curiosity within us with its awe-inspiring beauty and challenging terrain. The primal call that resonates with our ancient instincts is a testament to our intimate bond with Mother Nature. It reminds us, in silent whispers among rustling leaves or mighty roars of crashing waves, that we are creatures of this world — moulded by it, part of it, and forever tied to its ceaseless cycles.

Engaging in outdoor adventures comes as a return to our roots, our home away from the concrete jungles we've constructed. These activities offer an escape from our mundane routines, exposing us to the virtues of patience, serenity, resilience, and the raw thrill of standing against nature's fascinating caprices.

2.2. Facets of Outdoor Adventures

Outdoor adventures can take multiple shapes, each offering a unique set of challenges and experiences foregrounding nature's remarkable versatility.

Hiking and trekking through the undulating landscapes not only allow a leisurely encounter with nature but also provide a test of strength and endurance, as the terrain often switches between friendly plains to steep, demanding elevations. The roving hills, shadowed valleys, and towering piles work in symphony to reward the undeterred foot traveler with panoramas that take the breath away.

Canoeing and kayaking, on the other hand, introduce enthusiasts to the myriad mysteries of water bodies — be it serene lakes, twisting rivers, or the wide-open sea. The gentle bobbing of a canoe on a sunlit lake or the heart-pounding thrill of navigating a kayak through rapid rivers not only fuels the adrenaline rush but also cultivates a deep sense of connection and respect for the reigning water bodies.

Rock climbing, while demanding an immense level of physical strength and mental tenacity, offers an unparalleled vantage point to gaze upon the world. The ascension, with each hand and foothold calculated, every breath echoing against the cliff, transforms into a humbling experience reinforcing the magnitude and grandeur of nature's constructs.

2.3. The Essence of Adventure and the Role of Physical Fitness

However, the journey is not without its challenges. Physical fitness is a key component of venturing into outdoor activities. A robust body conditions us to face surprises, overcome obstacles, and appreciate the beauty that each venture has to offer. There is a certain merit in the struggle — a sense of achievement that transcends the physical exertion and weaves into the very fabric of our experience in the great outdoors. This joy of overcoming gravels of discomfort initiates a ripple effect in our lives, instilling a sense of confidence and capability that transcends beyond the natural terrain.

2.4. Role of Mental Well-being

Just as physical wellness is pivotal, the exploration of natural vistas brings along tranquility and peace, lending a positive impact on our mental well-being. The soothing murmur of a stream, the rustle of leaves underfoot, the birdsong in the early dawn, or the echo of our own heartbeat against mountainsides — these sensory experiences work as a salve, nurturing our mental health.

2.5. Outdoor Adventures & Sustainable Tourism

While revelling in the great outdoors, it's crucial that we pay heed to the principles of sustainable tourism. Nature is a generous host, but it's crucial that we, as guests, tread gently on her. Using biodegradable products, minimizing waste, respecting wildlife, and leaving no trace are the cardinal rules to ensure that the beauty of the parental playground remains unspoiled for generations to come.

As we delve into the world of outdoor adventures, we are reminded time and again about the captivating interplay of physical endurance, mental perseverance, and a harmonious existence with nature. This chapter may be seen as a prelude, coaxing you into the mesmerizing realm of the outdoors, enticing you to lace up your boots, ready your gear, and tap into the spirit of exploration. Remember, the journey ahead is an enthralling tale of the grandeur of nature met by human resilience — a gripping narrative that awaits your footprints. Stay with us as we dive deeper into this vast expanse, trailblazing our way into the heart of where the wild things are, fueled by earth's bountiful and nutritious provisions.

Chapter 3. The Importance of Nutrition in Outdoor Adventures

When it comes to outdoor adventures, the fusion of nature's embrace and your own bodily strength is truly serene. A large part of that strength comes from your nutrition, an aspect which is not to be overlooked. Nutrition serves as the foundation for any outdoor adventure, be it hiking, mountaineering or any other form of physical exertion.

3.1. Understanding the Connection

Outdoor activities frequently demand far more energy than everyday routines. From climbing intimidating slopes to crossing vigorous rivers, nature often poses tough yet enticing challenges. Navigating these takes a significant amount of energy. This is where adequate nutrition comes in, to ensure that your body is capable of meeting such demanding challenges. In order to maintain strength, stamina, and endurance, it is fundamental to consume energy-rich foods.

Think of your body as a complex machine. Just as a machine needs fuel to run, your body needs food to function. The nutrition you derive from your food is the very fuel that powers your body.

3.2. The Role of Macronutrients

There are three essential macronutrients that your body significantly requires for outdoor adventures: carbohydrates, proteins, and fats.

Carbohydrates are your body's main source of energy. During digestion, carbohydrates are broken down into glucose, which is used by your body's cells for energy. Depending upon their structure, carbohydrates can be classified into simple and complex carbohydrates. While simple carbohydrates provide instant energy, complex carbohydrates offer a prolonged supply. For demanding physical activities, it is advisable to ingest both types.

Proteins are the building blocks of your body. They not only help in muscle building and repair but also play a critical part in functions like transporting nutrients or forming antibodies. For outdoor adventurers, consuming a balanced amount of protein helps ensure muscle recovery post strenuous exercises.

Fats, though often looked down upon, are indispensable. They provide insulation, are fundamental for a host of bodily functions, and most importantly, serve as a sustained source of energy for long-lasting activities. Foods rich in unsaturated fats, such as avocados, nuts and seeds, provide energy and have added health advantages.

3.3. Hydration is Key

A glaring aspect of nutrition that is sometimes neglected – hydration. Water plays a crucial role in an abundance of physical processes like carrying nutrients and oxygen to cells, regulating body temperature, and flushing out toxins to name a few. When engaging in outdoor activities, your body loses much water through sweating, making it vital to intake ample quantities to stay hydrated.

3.4. Meal Planning Strategies

When planning meals for outdoor adventures, your goal should be to pack nutrient-dense foods that are lightweight and non-perishable. Opt for whole grains, dried fruits, nuts, seeds, and jerky, which provide abundant nutrition without carrying any excess weight.

A strategic technique for meal planning is to allocate your food intake throughout the day. Begin your day with a robust breakfast packed with complex carbohydrates and proteins for sustained energy and muscle function. Continue with snacks rich in both simple and complex carbohydrates for instant and prolonged energy. Finish with a high-protein recovery meal at the end of the day.

3.5. Wrapping it Up

Maintaining energy levels and optimal body function in the face of rigorous outdoor activities lies in efficient nutrition management. A firm understanding of your body's requirements and strategic meal planning is the key to achieving this.

To hike, swim, climb, paddle, or run in the great outdoors is an invigorating experience, one brimming with challenges and joys. As you dive deep into the wild, remember that the breath-taking landscapes and their challenges are only part of the adventure. The other part? It's the food you carry, the fuel that powers your journey. Hence, mindful nutrition is an absolute must. It is in this blend of nutrient-rich food and energizing activities that the essence of a rewarding outdoor adventure lies.

Chapter 4. Fueling the Adventure: A Look into Energy Foods

Our journey into the heart of outdoor adventures calls us to survey the engine that keeps the journey coursing: the very food that fuels our bodies. When embarking on outdoor adventures, energy-dense, lightweight, and easily packable food is a must. These foods not only support our physical exertion but also form a satisfying part of the experience, introducing us to new facets of taste and nutrition. Stepping into the wild calls for a diet plan that respects the primal roots of nourishment, marrying practicality with nutritional wisdom.

4.1. The Energy Demand of Outdoor Activities

Strenuous physical activities, such as hiking, mountain climbing, canoeing, demand an impressive supply of energy. Our bodies, comparable to intricate machines, require fuel to function, and the more intense the machine, the more fuel it burns. Experts estimate that backpacking can burn up to 600 calories per hour, depending on the weight of the backpack, trail difficulty, and the hiker's weight. This substantial demand for calories explains the need for energy-rich foods when you're challenging yourself under the open sky.

4.2. Essential Nutrients for Outdoor Activities

Like all machines, our bodies need more than just one type of fuel. In this regard, nutrients play different roles. There are three primary sources of energy - carbohydrates, protein, and fats. Carbohydrates are the primary source of immediate energy, proteins support muscle recovery and growth, and fats provide the highest amount of energy per gram, making it an efficient fuel source for long-term energy needs.

People often underestimate the importance of micronutrients such as vitamins and minerals. They boost immune functions, help repair bodily tissues, and facilitate the conversion of food into energy.

4.3. Favorite Energy Foods of Adventurers

Many outdoor adventurers have their favorites when it comes to 'energy' foods. Below is a list of go-to food items most often found in an adventurer's pack:

1. Nuts and Seeds: Almonds, walnuts, chia seeds, and flaxseeds pack a punch of protein, fiber, and healthy fats.

2. Nut Butter: Compact and bursting with protein and good fats, nut butter is handy for a quick energy boost.

3. Whole Grain Bread/Crackers: They're a great source of long-lasting carbohydrate energy.

4. Jerky: Beef or turkey jerky provides a protein-packed, non-perishable snack.

5. Dried Fruits: Raisins, apricots, dates and the likes offer a concentrated source of Quick carbohydrates along with vital minerals.

6. Dark Chocolate: A delicious indulgence filled with antioxidants, and it also provides a measured caffeine kick.

4.4. Energy Food Recipes for the Outdoors

While there are many ready-to-eat options available, it's also possible to prepare your own energy-packed food. Not only can this be cost-effective, but it also allows for customization according to individual preferences. Here are some simple to make outdoor food recipes:

4.4.1. Energy Bars

Energy bars are lightweight, non-perishable, and simple to consume on the go. A DIY energy bar allows for the incorporation of preferred ingredients:

Ingredients: . 1 cup of nuts . 1 cup of dried fruit . 1 cup of oats or rice barley Process: . Blend nuts in a food processor until they are in small pieces. Be careful not to blend them into a paste. . Incorporate oats into the mixture, followed by dried fruit. . Press the mixture into an 8-inch baking sheet, chill overnight, and cut into bars.

4.4.2. Peanut Butter Sandwich with a Twist

A classic peanut butter sandwich provides simple carbs, protein, and good fats. Plus, it is open to delightful augmentations:

Ingredients: . Whole-grain bread . Natural peanut butter . Dark chocolate chips or cacao nibs . Honey or agave syrup Process: . Spread a generous layer of peanut butter onto your bread. . Sprinkle dark chocolate chips or cacao nibs for a dose of antioxidants. . Drizzle with honey or agave syrup for additional natural sweetness.

4.5. H20: The Essential Element

In addition to food, water is the other crucial fuel for outdoor exercise. Staying hydrated helps regulate your body temperature, lubricates your joints, and aids in transporting nutrients to provide energy for your body. It is recommended to drink enough so that you're not thirsty and to maintain an almost light-color urine.

4.6. Beyond Nutrition

Finally, there's a psychological aspect to consider. Eating familiar and liked foods provide comforting, morale-boosting effects. Surviving on high-energy, but tasteless food could make a challenging trek less enjoyable. So it's not only about what gives the most energy, but also about how food choices affect the overall experience.

Just as with the outdoors, exploring the domain of energy foods calls for immersion, experience, and curiosity. So pack your backpack, bring along your favorite energy foods, and let nature be your guide.

Thus, through humankind's primal roots, we see the canvas where nutrition and adventure intertwine— giving birth to a unique and wonderful form of human experience, which is outdoors exploration. As you plan your next outdoor excursion, consider all aspects of energy foods - from calories to taste - and let your outdoor culinary adventure begin!

Chapter 5. Matching the Terrain: Tailoring Nutrition to Adventure Types

Adventure is a thrilling pursuit that calls forth our daring spirit, challenging us to put to test our physical and mental prowess. The diverse terrains that form the backdrop of outdoor adventures each have unique demands and require suitably tailored nourishment strategies. Equipping yourself with the right energy-dense foods becomes a crucial part of the adventure-planning. This chapter builds a clear link between the type of adventure and the kind of nutrition it requires.

5.1. Trekking in Mountains

Mountain trekking is a demanding exercise that requires vast amounts of energy to scale altitudes and trek across challenging terrains. High-energy eating is thus necessary to fuel your trekking expedition.

1. Carbohydrates: Being the body's primary source of energy, foods rich in carbohydrates are a must. Foods such as whole grain bread, oatmeal, bananas, and sweet potatoes are ideal.

2. Proteins: For muscle recovery and growth, consume proteins like nuts, beans, poultry, and fish.

3. Water: Keep yourself hydrated and prevent altitude sickness. Aim for hydrating foods such as fruits and vegetables in addition to regular water intake.

5.2. Canoeing and Kayaking

Canoeing and kayaking are full-body workouts that call for both strength and endurance. A balanced diet rich in carbohydrates, proteins and healthy fats will go a long way in powering your paddling expedition.

1. Carbohydrates: Whole grain pasta, brown rice, and quinoa provide sustained energy.

2. Proteins: Lean meats, tofu, eggs, and lentils are excellent choices.

3. Fats: Avocados, nuts and seeds provide healthy fats.

4. Snacks: Dried fruits and nuts, energy bars, and bananas can be munched through the day.

5.3. Desert Exploration

Desert exploration presents a set of unique challenges related to hydration and electrolyte balance. Eat water-rich foods and salty snacks to replenish lost fluids and salt.

1. Hydration: Carry drinking water, but also consider juicy fruits like watermelons and oranges.

2. Electrolytes: Snacks like pickles or electrolyte drinks aid in replenishing salt.

3. Energy: Trail mix, nuts, and energy bars are light-weight, non-perishable and provide quick energy.

5.4. Rock Climbing

Rock climbing demands high strength, endurance, and mental concentration. Frequent snacks rich in carbohydrates and protein will help restore energy and facilitate muscle recovery.

1. Carbohydrates: Energy bars, bananas, whole grain bread are easy to carry and rich in energy.

2. Proteins: A handful of nuts and seeds, a slice of lean meat or a hard-boiled egg can fulfill the required protein intake.

3. Hydration: Water is essential to prevent muscle cramps. Hydrating fruits can be included as well.

5.5. Arctic Adventures

In cold climates, your body burns more calories to maintain body temperature. Higher intakes of calorie-dense foods are required.

1. Carbohydrates & Fats: Calorie-dense foods like whole grains, fatty fish, nuts and seeds are great to keep the body energized.

2. Hydration: Staying hydrated is necessary even in cooler climates.

5.6. Jungle Safari

Jungle safaris require alertness and endurance. Light but nutritious meals throughout the day can keep you firing on all cylinders.

1. Carbohydrates: Fruits, nuts, and oats can be easily carried for sustained energy.

2. Proteins: Protein bars, nuts, cheese, or hard-boiled eggs fulfil protein requirements.

3. Water: Along with plenty of drinking water, include hydrating fruits and vegetables in your meal.

In conclusion, eating for an adventure involves understanding the physical rigors involved and consuming appropriately tailored nutrients. Regardless of the destination, always prioritize hydration and carry extra food than you think you might need. It's time to propel your outdoor adventures with nature's energy-boosting bounty!

Chapter 6. The Backpack Chef: Preparing Energy Foods in the Wild

Choosing the right food for your outdoor adventure can be equally as important as choosing your trail. Your food energy, after all, fuels the journey, offering nourishment for every arduous trek and energizing you for those tumultuous river crossings or uphill treks. In this section, we'll guide you on how to prepare nutritious, energy-packed meals from nature's bounty while on the go, even in the heart of the wilderness.

6.1. Gathering Your Tools

Every culinary adventure begins with the right tools, and wilderness cooking is no different. You'll want to pack smart, equipping yourself with the right cooking gear that's lightweight, multipurpose, and durable. Here's what you'll likely need:

- A lightweight backpacking stove and fuel

- Compact cookware like a pot or skillet

- Utensils (think spork instead of a separate spoon and fork to save space)

- A reliable knife for food prep

- Something to eat from, like a lightweight, reusable camping bowl or even a durable plastic container that can serve dual purposes storing food as well

- A source of fire, like a firestarter or waterproof matches

With these essentials, you'll be ready to start cooking delicious, energy-filled meals even in the wild backcountry.

6.2. Provisioning Creatively

Depending on your trip's duration, you'll want to thoroughly plan your meals and snacks. Focus on high-energy, non-perishable items that will keep well in your pack.

- Carbohydrates: Ideal sources are whole grain wraps or bagels that are less likely to be squished in your bag than loaves of bread. Think about dehydrated pasta or rice meals, too.

- Proteins: Tuna or chicken in vacuum packs work well, as do hard cheeses, nuts, and jerky.

- Fruits and Vegetables: Opt for sturdy options like apples or carrots. Dehydrated fruits like raisins, bananas, or apricots also offer a lighter and more durable choice.

Remember, you are not limited to only freeze-dried meals and energy bars.

6.3. Mastering the Art of Wild Cooking

Without the convenience of a fully equipped kitchen, cooking in the wild can seem daunting. But with a bit of creativity and preparation, you can turn campsite meals into one of the highlights of your trip.

1. Plan your meals. Breakfast might be a pre-packed bag of oatmeal mixed with a handful of nuts and dried fruit. For lunch, consider a wrap with hard cheese, salami, mustard, and a robust vegetable like a bell pepper or cucumber. Dinner could be a dehydrated meal, like pasta or rice with a side of vacuum-packed chicken or tuna.

2. Prep ahead. Consider pre-mixing your meals before the trip. For instance, break all the oatmeal packets open, combine them with

some dried fruits, nuts, and powdered milk in a resealable bag. All you'll need to do is add heated water for a quick and hearty breakfast.

3. Portion wisely. Vacuum-sealed or ziplocked bags are your friends when it comes to both saving space and keeping your food fresh. Repackaging food into meal-size portions can also reduce waste and make meal prep easier once you're out in the wild.

4. Learn to cook one-pot meals. Skill in preparing quick, nutritious one-pot meals can be a lifesaver. These are meals where all the ingredients cook together in one pot, allowing for an easier preparation and fewer dishes.

5. Cook meals in batches. Cook larger quantities and plan to have leftovers for next meals. This consolidated cooking will save you fuel and time.

6.4. Staying Hydrated

Water is essential, especially when exerting yourself on a trail. Always have a reliable means of purifying water whether it be via boiling, using water-purification tablets, or a filter. Hydrating with teas or electrolyte drink mixes can add a fun twist to your regular drinking water, just make sure to maintain sufficient plain water intake as well.

6.5. Cleanup and Waste Management

Leaving no trace behind includes tidying your cooking and eating area, properly disposing of food waste, and doing dishes. Consider eco-friendly, biodegradable soap for cleaning, and remember to wash dishes at least 200 feet away from any water source to limit the ecological impact.

With the right tools, a bit of planning, key nutritional insights, and some creativity, you'll have everything you need to be a gourmet chef in the wilderness. The joy of preparing your own meals under the open sky, powered by your portable stove, can transform the outdoor experience, connecting you further to nature and its nourishing potential.

Chapter 7. Eating on the Trail: Nutritious On-The-Go Meal Ideas

Eating on the trail is all about finding the perfect blend of convenience, nutrition, and lightweight packing. The sustenance we carry should power us through arduous treks, steep climbs, and long canoeing days yet remain light enough not to hinder our progress. First, let's delve into the motives that drive our nutritional choices on the trail, and afterward, present an array of meal ideas that are both tasty and energy-packed.

7.1. The Principles of Trail Nutrition

Fueling your body appropriately during adventurous endeavors is paramount. It's not just about satisfying your hunger, but picking foods that are rich in essential nutrients. High-energy, easily digestible, and protein-packed foods are ideal for outdoor adventurists.

Protein serves to repair your body's muscles and tissues, whilst carbohydrates provide quick and sustainable energy. It's also important to consume enough fiber for a healthy digestive system. Finally, including fats in your diet can give a slow, steady release of energy over a longer period.

⇒ Green leafy vegetables, fruits, grains, nuts, and seeds offer a good mix of these nutrients but might prove inconvenient on a trail in their natural form. Here, we learn how to adapt these foods to fit our outdoor pursuits.

7.2. Healthful Meal Ideas for Hikers

This section assembles a repertoire of meal ideas suitable for different stages of your outdoor adventure, from the energizing start to the rejuvenating ending.

7.3. Power Breakfasts

Start your morning with a powerful kick of nutrients to keep you going strong throughout the day.

1. Overnight Oats: Soak oats overnight with a protein source like Greek yogurt or nut butter, a sweetener such as honey or maple syrup, and your favorite fruits and nuts.

2. Banana and Nut Butter Wraps: Spread any nut butter over a whole grain wrap. Add slices of banana and a sprinkle of granola before rolling it up.

3. Chia Pudding: Mix chia seeds with milk or a non-dairy option, honey, and fruits of choice. Let it sit overnight.

7.4. Mid-Trail Lunches

Maintain your energy midday with high-protein options filled with whole grains and lean proteins. These are easy to carry and required minimal or no cooking.

1. Quinoa Salad: Pre-cooked quinoa mixed with a blend of fresh veggies, beans, and a hint of zest for a punchy flavor.

2. Tuna Pita Pockets: Carry canned tuna and whole grain pitas, along with some condiments. Assemble before eating to avoid sogginess.

3. Trail Mix: Combine peanuts, almonds, sunflower seeds, dried fruit, and chocolate pieces for an instant energy snack.

7.5. Sustaining Dinners

A satisfying dinner helps you replenish your energy stores and repair any muscle damage sustained during the day's activities.

1. Lentil and Rice Bowls: Carry pre-cooked lentils and rice. Add a pack of mixed vegetables, and you have a satisfying meal—a hot water bath can warm it up.

2. Instant Noodle Soup: Just-add-water types of noodle soups can be healthier by adding dehydrated veggies and lean meats.

3. Freeze-Dried Meals: There's a range of quality freeze-dried meals available that are nutritionally balanced and flavorful.

7.6. Energizing Snacks and Desserts

Hydration and quick energy snacks keep you sharp during exercises.

1. Protein Bars: These are portable and packed with proteins and carbs that make them ideal trail snacks.

2. Fresh Fruit: Apples and oranges travel well and offer you a fresh, juicy break during your hike.

3. Dark Chocolate: A great source of antioxidants, and given its high-fat content, it's a sustainable source of energy too.

Understanding the nutritional needs of your body and the limitations posed by outdoor pursuits gets you half-prepared for your adventure. The other essential part is equipping yourself with nutritious food options that also taste great to keep your spirits high on the trail. This blend of nutritional wisdom and culinary creativity is the secret to uninterrupted outdoor exploration, uniting nature and nutrition in a delightful symphony.

Chapter 8. Foraging 101: Learning from Nature's Pantry

Peering into the verdant wilderness, we uncover nature's secret pantry, an abundant resource for those who dare to step off the beaten path. Foraging can turn a simple hike or camping trip into an exploratory journey of taste, nutrition, and survival skills. Rooted in our ancestral past, it's an art that goes hand-in-hand with outdoor adventures, a complementary skill to climbing, abseiling, rafting, or the gentle amble of a woodland walk. This chapter is your guide to gaining an eclectic mix of knowledge, part naturalist and part culinary, to bring your outdoor experience to another level.

8.1. Digging into History

Looking at the path that brought us here, our reliance on foraging has dwindled due to agricultural and industrial advances. However, the value of this skill goes beyond survival. It bridges the gap between human and landscape, entertaining, educating, and feeding us along the journey. Far from being a relic of the past, foraging encourages a closer bond with the very wilderness we appreciate and protects its diverse, delicate ecosystems through our careful interaction.

8.2. Essential Foraging skills

Being successful in foraging requires more than knowing which berries to pick. It's about knowing how and when to forage, alongside a sound understanding of the environment.

- **Identifying plants**: Knowledge of harmful and beneficial plants is paramount. Educing smooth and downy birch trees and burdock from elder and giant hogweed can create a pantry filled with nuts, roots, and sap which can be turned into delicious and nutritious meals.

- **Seasonal foraging**: Every season, nature offers different bounties. Knowing when to forage for what will maximize your yield.

- **Foraging ethics**: As a forager, you have a responsibility to protect the ecosystem you take from. Following the 'Leave No Trace' practice, taking only what you need, and understanding local laws and guidelines will ensure sustainable foraging.

8.3. Safety & Preparation

Before you start foraging, be prepared with suitable outdoor gear such as durable gloves to protect your hands, a basket or bag for your haul, a plant identification guide or app, and a small shovel or knife for digging and cutting.

As part of your safety routine, adhere to "The Forager's Rule of Three" – never consume anything unless you're 100% sure it's edible by cross-verifying with at least three reliable sources.

8.4. Guided Foraging Adventure

For beginners, joining a guided foraging adventure is a wise step. These excursions offer hands-on knowledge about the local biosphere, provide guidance on reading the land, and teach you how to identify plants correctly.

8.5. Making Meals

Freshly foraged ingredients can be put to great use. From simple salads and stir-fries to cordials, jams, and even beers, your creativity is the only limit. Remember that many wild foods are more nutritionally dense than their cultivated counterparts, adding that extra burst of energy on your venture.

8.6. The Bountiful Nutrition

From Stinging Nettles, a rich source of vitamins and minerals, to Blackberries, with their high antioxidant content, foraged foods are nutritional powerhouses. Understanding and harnessing these health benefits is a transformative phase in your foraging journey.

8.7. Forage for a Cause

As a forager, you have the potential to participate in citizen science projects such as monitoring the spread of invasive species or tracking the impact of climate change on local plant communities. Your exploration can contribute to large-scale environmental conservation and research initiatives.

To conclude, foraging is not just about food. It is a holistic practise fostering a greater connection with nature, understanding of ecological systems, and satiating our inherent curiosity. As we delve into this activity, we learn survival skills, appreciate the beauty of nature more authentically, and engage in preservation efforts.

Chapter 9. Food Safety: Keeping Your Outdoor Meals Fresh and Clean

Maintaining food safety is a critical aspect of any outdoor adventure. The value of a delicious, energy-packed meal can be quickly overshadowed by the consequences of foodborne illnesses if proper care and precautions aren't taken.

9.1. Understanding Foodborne Illnesses

Foodborne illnesses, commonly known as food poisoning, are caused by eating food contaminated with bacteria, parasites, viruses, or toxins. These illnesses can . occur when food isn't stored or prepared properly. Symptoms can be mild, like nausea and diarrhea, or severe, leading to dehydration, fever, or in extreme cases, hospitalization.

When you're out adventuring, a bout of food poisoning is more than just a discomfort. It can ruin an exciting trip, as it potentially puts your body under stress and impedes you from engaging in various activities.

9.2. Kit Essentials: Storage and Cooking Devices

For any outdoor escapade, having proper storage and cooking devices is the first step towards maintaining food safety.

1. **Insulated cooler**: An insulated cooler is crucial for keeping perishable food cold and reducing bacterial growth. Look for a

high-quality cooler that can maintain a temperature of below 40°F.

2. **Thermometer**: A reliable food thermometer helps ensure safe cooking and storage temperatures. It is particularly useful when cooking meats.

3. **Cooking Equipment**: Stoves, grills, or camping ovens are necessary for cooking food thoroughly and killing harmful bacteria.

4. **Water Purification System**: In addition to food, clean water is paramount. Use filtering systems, boiling, or purification tablets to ensure the water you consume is safe.

9.3. Safe Food Storage

Storing food correctly is critical in preventing foodborne illnesses. Bacteria multiplies rapidly between 40°F and 140°F, a danger zone where food spoilage accelerates.

Keep perishable foods like meats, dairy products, and prepared meals in a cooler until you're ready to cook. It's best to pack them already chilled or frozen. Store food in sealable plastic containers or bags to prevent cross-contamination.

Non-perishable items like dry food and canned goods should also be stored well. Keep them shielded from sunlight, and as cool as possible. Use airtight containers to protect your food from pests and moisture.

9.4. Safe Water Storage

Water that's safe for drinking is as critical as safe food. Store drinking water separate from dish or hand-washing water. If drawing water from a natural source, always assume it's unpure. Even crystal-clear, cold water can be full of microorganisms.

Boiling is the most reliable method to make water safe; keep the water boiling for at least a minute. If boiling isn't possible, use a water filter or purifying tablets as directed by the manufacturer.

9.5. Meal Preparation in the Outdoors

The outdoor environment is certainly different from your home kitchen. Remember the following pointers:

1. **Planned Cooking**: Chalk out your meal plan before the trip to minimize food handling. Prep ingredients, marinate meats, and wash fruits and vegetables beforehand.

2. **Safe Handling**: Always wash hands before and after handling food. Carry a hand sanitizer for times when you don't have access to warm water and soap.

3. **Avoid Cross-contamination**: Separate utensils and cutting boards should be used for raw and cooked food to prevent cross-contamination.

4. **Cooking Temperature**: Use a food thermometer to ensure cooked food reaches the required internal temperature for safety.

5. **Leftovers**: Promptly store leftovers in the cooler. If you doubt the safety of any food, remember: "When in doubt, throw it out!"

9.6. Safe Trash Disposal

Proper trash disposal prevents attracting animals and respects nature. Ensure all food wastes are collected and packed out of the campsite.

Following the guidelines in this chapter will ensure you stay healthy and allows you to truly enjoy the pinnacle of outdoor adventures. Freedom and exploration never tasted so good!

Chapter 10. Case Studies: Thriving against Elements with the Right Fuel

The numerous stories of outdoorsmen and women thriving against the elements, thanks to their balanced and energy-rich diets, are ample testament to the integral role that quality nutrition plays in such endeavours. Let's peek into their sagas, understand their choices, and the reasons behind them. Then, we can harness this wisdom to plot our own outdoor adventures. The individual ventures described here elucidate how preparation, adequate nutrition, and a deep respect for nature can lead to successful expeditions under varying circumstances.

10.1. First Case: Mike Leary, the Arctic Survivor

Our first subject is Mike Leary, an experienced mountaineer, who undertook a 30-day winter trek in the harsh terrains of the Arctic Tundra. With temperatures plummeting down to -40 degrees Celsius and unpredictable weather changes, Mike's adventure was incredibly challenging yet exhilarating.

Initially, Mike struggled with rapid exhaustion and dizziness, but he soon realised the importance of carving out a diet that maintained his energy levels and provided warmth. His diet primarily consisted of high-energy snacks like energy bars, trail mix, jerky and cheese, with a focus on consuming lots of fats due to their high calorific content.

Food	Reason for Inclusion
Energy Bars	Dense source of energy, easy to eat without preparation
Trail Mix	A mixture of nuts, seeds and sometimes chocolate provides a perfect balance of fat, protein, and carbohydrates
Jerky	High-protein snack, contributes to muscle recovery
Cheese	High in calories and fat, providing sustained energy and warmth

Mike's adventure underscores two crucial points: energy density matters, especially in harsh conditions, and that tweaking the diet to suit the environment aids survival.

10.2. Second Case: Emma White, the Long-distance Swimmer

Crossing the English Channel isn't a walk in the park. Emma White, a long-distance professional swimmer, undertook this daunting task. An open sea greeted Emma with water temperatures averaging 15 degrees Celsius, amidst strong tides and sea currents. It's a challenge as much about surviving the cold as it is about endurance.

Emma swam for an average of fourteen hours. Her diet needed to quickly replenish the energy lost and help maintain body temperature. Sports gels and isotonic drinks, rich in carbs and electrolytes, were her chosen nutrition during breaks, along with some warming soup and protein-rich shakes.

Food	Reason for Inclusion
Sports Gels	Compact and quick source of carbohydrates
Isotonic Drinks	Replenishes electrolytes, maintains hydration
Soup	Provides warmth, nourishment and easy to digest
Protein Shakes	Helps in muscle recovery and repair

Emma's journey serves as an example of tailored nutrition aiding in endurance activities, and underlines the importance of hydration and muscle recovery.

10.3. Third Case: Max Li, the Desert Explorer

Max Li, an intrepid explorer, opted for the parched expanse of the Sahara for his latest adventure. The scorching sun, arid environment, and constant need for hydration made his journey incredibly challenging.

Max needed a diet rich in slow-release carbohydrates to maintain energy levels, and one that minimises thirst arousal. He relied on dried fruits, nuts, and energy bars, along with rehydration salts to maintain his electrolyte balance.

Food	Reason for Inclusion
Dried Fruits	High in fibre, and offers slow-release energy
Nuts	Healthy fats, also provide sustained energy

Food	Reason for Inclusion
Energy Bars	Easy source of energy, doesn't induce thirst
Rehydration Salts	For maintaining electrolyte balance, crucial in desert environment

Max's experience mirrors the modified dietary requirements in a desert environment and teaches us the invaluable lesson of hydration in such settings.

In conclusion, these case studies serve as vivid illustrations of the role nutrition plays in outdoor adventures. The lessons learnt emphasize the need for manipulating the diet based on various factors, inclusive of weather conditions, physical exertion and the landscape one encounters. Adventurous souls must indeed brave the elements and the unknown terrains, but they mustn't forget to fuel their bodies adequately. Armed with knowledge, they'll find that nature, nutrition, and the human spirit can come together in an exhilarating, unstoppable brew.

Chapter 11. Embracing the Future: The Confluence of Adventure and Nutrition

From the dawn of time, adventure and nutrition have galloped together, shaping our evolution and paving the path of human prosperity. Adventure may look different in today's world compared to the pioneering times: fewer wild frontiers to discover, less untamed wilderness to conquer. Yet, the spirit of outdoor exploration endures, it has merely morphed into a modern-day quest for thrilling experiences engirdled by nature's serenity. In a similar vein, the science of nutrition has seen a tectonic shift. Ancient man's simple, survival-oriented food habits have spiraled into a sophisticated understanding of diet, energy consumption, and peak performance. The harmonious convergence of adventure and nutrition, then, holds the promise of a future where physical exploits are fuelled by intelligent and science-backed nutrition.

11.1. The Enthralling Alliance

Our bodies need fuel to function, especially in physically demanding activities such as mountain biking, rock climbing, hiking, or kayaking. It turns out, though, that not all food is created equal. The energy density, satiety, ease of digestion, and nutrient profile of different foods can greatly impact performance and endurance. Also, during outdoor adventures, practical considerations such as weight, packability, and spoilage are paramount importance. Whether fresh-caught fish roasted over a campfire or sophisticated energy bars packed with protein and complex carbohydrates, each type of food serves a distinct purpose.

11.2. The Rise of Adventure Nutrition

Nutrition for outdoor endeavors used to be a relatively simple affair built around convenience and availability : canned beans, hardtack, and jerky. In time though, outdoor enthusiasts started understanding the importance of nutrition, launching a seismic shift in adventure food. Energy bars, hydration tablets, isotonic drinks, and high-protein meals have invaded the adventurer's pack, all designed to provide optimal nutrition while minimizing pack weight and maximizing shelf-life. Evolutions in cooked meals as well, such as the advent of dehydrated food packs and ready-to-eat meals, means that outdoor enthusiasts can now enjoy more varied, nutritious, and palate-pleasing menus during their wilderness sorties.

11.3. The Science of Performance Foods

Performance matters immensely in outdoor adventures. That's where performance nutrition comes into the picture. Energy-dense foods that are easily digestible and can be consumed on the go are just the tip of the iceberg. We're now witnessing a rise in research surrounding dietary supplements and modifications aimed at boosting athletic performance. Beta-alanine, creatine, caffeine - we are certainly a far cry from the humble can of beans. However, these aren't off-the-shelf magic pills; when done right, these science-backed nutritional strategies require a good understanding of their interactions with the body and continuous adjustments in response to individual needs and outcomes.

11.4. Fueling Up for Outdoor Challenges

Choosing the right food is a delicate balancing act. Physiologically, there has to be a proper ratio of macro nutrients – carbohydrates, proteins, and fats, as well as a host of essential micronutrients (the vitamins and minerals). This needs to be tailored to the physical demands of the adventure. For instance, high-intensity activities demand a greater proportion of carbohydrates for immediate energy demands, while moderate to low-intensity, or long-duration activities might need slow-burning fats to back endurance. The body requires protein for recovery and muscle building, so that should factor into the dietary planning as well.

11.5. Nourishing the Adventurer's Spirit

All work and no play makes Jack a dull boy. The old adage holds true even for nutrition. While function might be paramount while planning adventure foods, enjoyment is a close second. To keep the spirits high and the body's hearth stoked, the food must nourish the soul just as it feeds the muscle. That's why the likes of hot cocoa and s'mores still delight, and likely will continue to, modern-day adventurers.

Evidently, the future lies at the crossroads of these two incredible pursuits. The cutting edge of research continues to decode the intimate relationship between our bodies and our diet, and how best to harness that knowledge for the adventurer's advantage, thus promising the realization of an exciting future where nutrition and adventures are two sides of the same coin. Outdoor enthusiasts of the future can look forward to scaling the frontier between physical prowess and nutritional wisdom with an impeccably packed rucksack of scientifically backed food products. Indeed, it seems that the bond between adventure and nutrition is only poised to grow stronger, driving us further into the arms of nature with health and vitality.